A Taste of Our Own Medicine

3 Vital Keys to Ending Postnatal Depletion,
Nurturing Mothers, and Improving Communities

Danett C. Bean, DAAM

Disclaimer
This book contains information that is intended to help the reader become a better-informed consumer of health care. It is not intended as a substitute for the medical advice of a physician. The reader should consult with a doctor in any matter related to her/his health. Always consult your doctor for your individual needs.

MESSAGE TO READERS

This book is interactive! All of the QR (Quick Response) codes throughout the book can be scanned with your smartphone or tablet to watch the accompanying videos.

How to Scan the QR Codes in This Book

Step 1: Download a free QR Code Reader onto your smartphone by searching the App Store. I selected the Kaywa Reader because it is free of advertisements.

Step 2: Tap the app once it has downloaded to your phone; this will open up the reader. Tap again, and your camera will appear to be on. Hover over the code you wish to scan, and the camera will automatically take a picture of the QR code; then your phone will be directed to the respective web page on backtothemiddle.com that contains each video message.

Here are some free tools to help improve the health of mothers and women:

Your free Postnatal Care Template
**http://backtothemiddle.com/
postnatal-care-checklist-freebie/**

5 Minutes of Energetic Recharge for Total Women's Health video
**http://backtothemiddle.com/5-minutes-of-
energetic-recharge-for-total-womens-health-video/**

Your free Fibroid Prevention Guide
**http://backtothemiddle.com/
fibroid-prevention-guide/**

Dedicated to my mother, and all of the mothers known and unknown who have given their blood, bone, and vital essence to sustain us all and to keep the world moving. To those mothers gone too soon: Sabira Abdullah, Lynn Best, Constance Bean, Aqa Aakhu Mothudi, Faybiene Miranda, and all those that have not been mentioned.

To our daughters, granddaughters, and future generations who prayerfully will live in a world where they always give from a full cup.

Table of Contents

"While childbearing women and programs and policies for them focus extensively on care during pregnancy and around the time of birth, considerably less attention is given to women's postpartum health, including access to high-quality care and coordinated services after birth. However, postpartum maternal health influences women's lifetime risk of chronic disease, health in subsequent pregnancies, family functioning, and the well-being of children and other family members **(Childbirth Connection, 2017).**"

CHAPTER 1

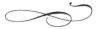

What Is Postnatal Depletion?

Watch Video Message:
Danett C. Bean, DAAM Introduces Chapter 1
http://backtothemiddle.com/a-taste-of-our-own-medicine-book-chapter-1-introduction-video/

I didn't know where I was. I blinked my eyes. I saw folders and all kinds of stationary. The light was halogen. Straight ahead there were people working behind registers. I looked to my left and saw past glass doors. It was night out. I had to concentrate because the one thing I knew was that I wasn't home, and somehow I needed to get there and get to my baby. *"Focus Danett"*, I kept telling myself. *"Why am I here?"* If I could figure that out then maybe it could help me to get home. Somehow, I made my way out of the door and tried to find a taxi.

This wasn't the first time I'd felt this way, nor would it be the last. In addition to sometimes not knowing where I was,

I'd often feel so tired. My left wrist had gone out, to the point that sometimes it was hard to hold my baby boy. Since having him, I'd had a long list of ailments including repeated MRSA episodes, thirteen cavities that I didn't have before pregnancy, a lupus diagnosis, and a host of other ailments. So please pardon the energy that it took not to laugh in the faces of those who dared to ask when the second baby was coming.

I'd hoped that as my son got older things would get better, but for a while they didn't. His energy picked up and mine slowed down. I remember looking at his face and loving him so much. His face is so beautiful and his zest for life is so palpable, but there were days that I dreaded our time together for fear of not being able to keep up with him. I felt terrible. We made it, but it was really hard. Really hard.

One of my health practitioners had suggested that I reduce my already-reduced work hours, but it was difficult because we needed the money. We had to dip into the money that my husband and I had saved for maternity leave to move to a new apartment. Our prior landlord wanted to use chemicals in our apartment that were dangerous for fetal development. We ended up making an unplanned move when I was seven months pregnant.

My husband was doing the best that he could, but he was often upset about doing housework that we were behind in. We had so many intense disputes, and there was so much silence. Our relationship suffered tremendously. Things were frequently so tense that I really didn't know if we would make it. We have been together many years, but had never had such a rough patch. I tried talking to him about it, but what my husband didn't understand was that more times than not I didn't feel well, even if I looked like I did. He also didn't realize that I was struggling in every area of my life. I was drowning, and drowning quickly, but I didn't know what to do about it.

One day a friend sent me a link to http://goop.com/postnatal-depletion-even-10-years-later/ and asked me to check it out. I read the article by Dr. Oscar Serrallach, and for the first time in a long time I felt a little bit of hope. While I had wonderful health practitioners, some of them just seemed to believe that I was going through a "rough stretch." Without their help, I'm certain that I wouldn't still be here. Still, hearing a name for my diagnosis made something inside me feel better, and made me feel less crazy. As a health practitioner myself, this gave me insight into what it must be like for my patients. There is an ease that comes across their faces when they finally have some way to categorize their experience.

I recall the midwife that discharged me from the hospital. She told me to take it really slow, and reminded me that I had been through a lot. She was referring to the significant amount of blood loss I'd had and the fourth-degree tear I had experienced giving birth (If you don't know what a fourth-degree tear is, be glad. It's a complete tear of the perineum from the vagina to the anus. Yeah ouch!!!). I took her words in as much as I could, but I didn't know how to translate that into my life.

Because this was my first child and I had little to no informa-tion, I thought I *was* taking it easy. It turns out that what she was warning me about was postnatal depletion.

Postnatal depletion, also referred to as depleted mother syn-drome (DMS), postpartum nutritional depletion, or postpar-tum fatigue/exhaustion, is a collection of health issues that mothers may experience after giving birth. From a standpoint of traditional Asian medicine, which I am formally trained in, postnatal depletion can be classified as a form of taxation fatigue. Symptoms can include memory disturbances, dif-ficulty concentrating, emotional fluctuations, fatigue, joint issues, autoimmune and thyroid conditions, etc. As mothers, we can naturally be tuned in with our babies' needs; however, if we become "hypervigilant", and without sufficient support, this can be harmful to the mother (Serallach, n.d.). That defi-nitely explained my experience: –1000 energy on a scale of 1 to 10, the times that I didn't know where I was, and the other symptoms I had.

I'd heard that "pregnancy brain" could continue through nursing. But my symptoms had continued *past* nursing. Even though my goal had been to give my son the option of nursing until he was two years old, an intense MRSA episode caused me to be put on antibiotics, and so we had to stop nursing ear-lier than I had planned. I think I was more upset about it than he was. The one condition that I had heard of that mothers might experience after giving birth was postpartum depres-sion. It turns out that postnatal depletion can actually cause postpartum depression, and vice versa. So it is quite possible that some cases of postpartum depression may actually be postnatal depletion, or related to it.

Oftentimes, it seems like the importance of maternal health vanishes as the baby leaves the body after giving birth, and the effects on the mother after this huge miraculous event are nonexistent. It's like you're supposed to just snap back into shape and function as though nothing had ever happened. If that's your story that is absolutely wonderful! Thumbs up! But for myself and the estimated 50% of women affected by postnatal depletion, that's not our story.

Many times as new mothers, we can get caught up in how close our labor came to how we had planned for it to happen. I truly believe that even with the high rates of unnecessary medical interventions during birth, even if your birth story isn't what you envisioned, it is perfect because a new life—from what I believe to be the highest source there is—came through you. Whether that baby came through the front door, back door, or window, his or her arrival is perfect and that work of mothers should be left intact, as opposed to being the subject of scrutiny, as can often happen.

Losing My Mind

There were times that I felt like I was losing my mind. In retrospect, I believe that this was largely due to feeling overwhelmed and frustrated, along with whatever else accompanies you when you have a big job to do, but not the fuel to back it up. It was like trying to press hard on the gas pedal in a car without gas. The other part was that I *had* lost some of my mind, or rather my brain, as mothers' brains actually shrink 5% in the prenatal period, to support the baby's growth and to prepare our minds for the next phase of the journey of motherhood. This is another way of mother nature and the intelligence of our bodies. So while this part of the beautiful work of motherhood happened by nature's design, I don't believe that to be true about the other aspects of postnatal depletion. And what about the factors that could predispose you to postnatal depletion? From my own personal experience, and as someone who has specialized in women's health for many years, I've gathered the following as potential contributing factors.

1. Fat and Nutrient Loss

A lot of fat and nutrient loss happens during the last term of pregnancy. There are reasons why you may not be keeping up with your additional dietary requirements. In my case, we had to move so I was caught up in packing and making sure that we had a home in which to deliver our baby, since we were planning a home birth. My son was also born in August during a typical hot and humid New York summer. The weather, combined with my darling burner that I was carrying around with me, did not make me particularly hungry.

2. The Type of Labor and Birth

Tears of the perineum, such as the one that I experienced, can also contribute to postnatal depletion. From a traditional Asian medical standpoint, there is an important channel or energy pathway that passes through the perineum called the conception vessel. It contains a type of energy that is important to the vitality of the body. It also passes through the midline of the front of the body, so for those that have had a cesarean, this can play a role as well. A lot of blood loss can also be a factor, as I can attest to. In traditional Asian medical theory, blood is considered to be a precious substance. A loss of this substance can directly lead to a depletion of *qi*, or energy, which can make it more challenging for the body to carry out and/or maintain some of its basic functions.

3. Postnatal Life

If your postnatal life was like that of women in many indigenous cultures, it was probably pretty good compared to a lot of ours. In places like Korea and China, for example, for the first month following labor, the mother just rests and nurses the baby (in China this is referred to as *zuo yue zi*, or "sitting the month"). If that wasn't your experience, I can relate. My postnatal life was mainly my husband, myself, and baby, with hardly any additional support. There was also financial stress that caused me to return to work sooner than what would've been ideal. Pressure, stress, and strife can definitely negatively affect postnatal life and contribute to postnatal depletion.

Of note is the fact that many women are already depleted going into pregnancy. But why are some women already depleted before they become pregnant? There are a variety of reasons as to why this might be.

1. Stress and Trauma

We all know what stress is. What's important is to have a good self-care regimen in place. This should include physical exercise that you enjoy at least three times a week, some healthy and consistent way of processing emotions, and being a part of some community. Having some relationship to a higher power, God, or how you understand the source of things to be, and a whole foods-based diet are also important components.

Traumas are significant events that happen in our lives that are deeply distressing. Many of us have had such events and are aware of them, while for others the traumas get buried deep into a place far out of our conscious. From a traditional Asian medical standpoint, stress and trauma can impact the energy flow in the body, which in large amounts can wreak havoc on the body. The effects of this can directly or indirectly lead to depletion. I have dealt with both stress and trauma over the years, and I've found that this can be very draining unless one is able find a positive perspective (i.e., getting the lesson from the stress or trauma, and using that lesson for healing).

2. Lifestyle

Lifestyle can be a factor in being depleted prior to becoming pregnant. From a traditional Asian medical standpoint, choices that we make—particularly about different substances that we put in our bodies—can affect what is referred to as *jing*. *Jing* can be understood as a key substance that controls the aging process and vitality, which can affect overall health and reproductive health. Caffeine is a common substance that depletes *jing*. When we consume caffeine it can seem like we're getting so much energy, but some traditional Asian medical theories state that this feeling is actually using our *jing*, or health and energy reserves. It's like having a credit card and going on a spending spree without realizing that you will have to pay this money back.

Other common substances that may be part of one's lifestyle, like nicotine and alcohol, can also be depleting. Diet, beverages, what you put in and around your body (including drug use), how you spend your time, and how your life is set up are all a part of lifestyle. If set up well, your lifestyle can enhance your health, or at least help you to maintain it. If not, it can lead to health complications, including depletion. If a woman has regularly encountered stress, such as stress from school, career, a partner, or a family member that causes drama that they have internalized, this can be depleting. It is also important to consider a term that in traditional Asian medical theory is called overwork. Overwork can be a factor in illness, and it is just what it sounds like: working too much, exceeding what is healthy for the body. Drawing from my own experiences, I have overextended myself in different ways over the years. If not kept up with, your health account can surely become overdrawn.

One very important aspect of lifestyle is sleep. Sleep is a thing in and of itself. It is such an important activity, and there is still much research to be done in this area. Many of us have burned the midnight oil preparing for exams in college or hanging out at the club. But as we get older, late nights can catch up. Particularly in my private practice, I've noticed how depleted people who work nights can become—primarily because it throws off their circadian rhythm. Many jobs pay higher rates for night shift workers, and everyone does what they have to do. It is important to note, however, that even with the extra much-needed income, we still can end up paying with our health.

2. Age

Age is an interesting factor. As we get older, our body systems and functions tend to decline, unless we are living an excellent lifestyle, and or have exceptional genes. It is interesting because this also comes back to *jing*. Our *jing* directly affects our aging process. So a woman who is 31 and was not born with a high quality of jing, and has had a lot of stress and trauma while living an unhealthy lifestyle, can be depleted. Whereas a woman of 40 who has not experienced a lot of trauma and has had a healthy lifestyle in place (including a good self-care and stress management regimen), and who was born with higher quality jing, may be less depleted than the 31-year-old woman.

Regardless of whether a woman was depleted prior to pregnancy or not, postnatal depletion can still occur due to the type of labor and birth she had, and to lack of support she received postnatally. The stresses of daily living, including finances and many other factors, can also play a role. Postnatal depletion can be devastating and set the stage for other health issues. I believe it is possible to end postnatal depletion, and this is the very thing that we discuss in the next chapter.

CHAPTER 2

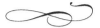

How Do We End Postnatal Depletion?

Watch Video Message:
Danett C. Bean, DAAM Introduces Chapter 2
http://backtothemiddle.com/a-taste-of-our-own-medicine-book-chapter-2-introduction-video/

To end postnatal depletion we must assist those who currently have it, and set up the conditions to prevent it from occurring in the future. To do this we must look back at history, as understanding the past can definitely help to change the future.

How Did We Get Here?

Many indigenous cultures around the world have certain customs that exist, and have existed for a long time, that naturally provide mothers with high-quality postnatal care.

I have lived all of my life in the United States of America, mainly in the city of New York. New York is a huge melting pot of amazing cultures. However, for those who move here and assimilate into American culture, it is important to maintain ties to one's culture and postnatal traditions. For example, one patient who came to me for prebirth treatments was of Dominican heritage. When we discussed her postnatal care plan, she told me that her mother already had the hens to make her a traditional soup. This patient had a great postnatal recovery. There are many factors that went into her successful recovery, but I believe the nourishing foods from her heritage were key. As an African American who is still researching the roots of my ancestral traditions, I have begun to create some of my own soup (See resource section, Things That Personally Helped Me to Recover from Postnatal Depletion).

Regardless of ancestry, many women in this country have been told that the newer Western medical approach to pregnancy and birth is better than the traditional approach of indigenous cultures, and that it is necessary to accept this model if you want the best for your baby. I am very much an advocate of patient-centered medicine, using any and all medical practices that are most helpful to the patient and her health—physically, emotionally, and spiritually. Many indigenous peri-birth practices seem to be centered in assisting a woman to trust in her innate female intuition, while Western medical practices shine in true cases of emergency. Perhaps one day peri-birth care in this country will be inclusive of the best that each system of medicine has to offer, and will be provided as standard integrative care for mothers, families, and individuals alike.

Capitalism

While capitalism has created numerous positive gains, such as easier access to basic human survival for many (but definitely not all) of us, there have also been negatives. These include the increased need for many people to work long hours to keep up with the cost of living and its demands. The amount of time that many people are forced to work has not allowed for maternity and paternity leave as a standard. It has caused more women and their partners to return to work sooner after having a baby than they would have chosen otherwise. This was certainly true for my husband and I.

Many of us in the United States, particularly city dwellers, can attest to this hamster wheel way of life. Lots of us struggle just to keep up with basic demands, and many of those with money don't have time. These factors make it harder for community to happen naturally, which has resulted in a greater shift toward individuality and the nuclear family.

Ending Postnatal Depletion

There are cultures around the world that have figured out how to support mothers and families in the postnatal period. In Mexico and Germany this precious time is recognized. In Asia, it is called *zouyuzei*, in the Netherlands *kraamzorg*. Societies with high quality postnatal care ingrained into their culture seem to mimic that which the mother is providing for the baby:

1. Sleep/Rest
2. Nutritious foods
3. Peace and solace

A significant part of ending postnatal depletion is to further postnatal care. For mothers, this is a taste of our own medicine, where we are set up to receive all the aspects of care that are required to sustain a new life. If it takes a village to raise a child, it must at least take a smaller village to help sustain those that incubate and develop the child.

The following three ingredients also seem to be inherent in cultures with high-quality postnatal care:

1. Acknowledgment of the need for postnatal care
2. Community
3. Support

To end postnatal depletion, we must further postnatal care in 21st century America, as well as all places in the world where postnatal depletion occurs. These three ingredients—acknowledgement of postnatal care, community, and support—are essential to begin this process. Each will be discussed in the upcoming chapters, followed by a proposal for the future and a resource section on:

- A letter, "For the Mother Who Thinks She May Have Postnatal Depletion"
- Helpful tips to support mothers
- Postnatal Care template checklist
- A quick list of what helped me to recover

It is my deep desire to end stories like mine, and to help other mothers and families have a higher quality of life. To strengthen postnatal care, we must first acknowledge it.

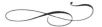

Acknowledgment

Watch Video Message:
Danett C. Bean, DAAM Introduces Chapter 3
http://backtothemiddle.com/a-taste-of-our-own-medicine-book-chapter-3-introduction-video/

Like many hard things, acknowledgment begins the healing—without it, not much can be done. The question after that becomes, "*How* do we heal?"

There are numerous reasons why acknowledgment of postnatal care has often been skipped in the United States, far more than what can be covered in the scope of this book. From my observations and research, I believe that the role of women in this country plays a huge part. I also believe that we are generally focused on the product and not the process, similar to the idea of fast food. So in a sense, the results are often rendered complete and separate from their origination and process. Couple this with sexism, and it's easy to see how postnatal care has been limited. Sexism has been, and continues to be, a topic that not everyone believes exists. Like all the -isms, if you have not experienced it, it may very well not exist to you. Or, if you are a part of that group and your eyes aren't open to it, you may miss it. Like a fish constantly swimming in water, it is not easy to describe that which we are constantly submersed in.

Many additional factors exist. For example, some older generations feel that since they didn't have help, mothers don't need this assistance and will figure it out. And we do figure it out, but at what expense? It is seen as sort of a sick initiation into parenting, but anytime we purposely do not assist the mother with a child, the mother suffers, the child suffers, and the family suffers. This suffering and sickness continues to be passed on through the generations, which is limiting and unnecessary. I believe that in part, the roots of this may come from long histories in which women have had to struggle on no matter what, particularly based on race and class. There are positives and negatives that can arise from such events. Resilience and resourcefulness are positives, but having lower expectations, becoming numb to those expectations, and settling into an attitude of "that's just the way it is" are negatives. Just because a group knows how to struggle on, does that tradition need to continue, especially if more resources are available? I don't think so. I think this tradition of letting mothers and families struggle and suffer is past its usefulness, and has now become detrimental to current and future generations. It's good to give what you didn't have; not just what you think someone should have, but what is actually needed, if you are able to.

Still many others just don't think about it, don't even realize that there's something going on, or that this needs to be acknowledged. Many mothers have become so accustomed to the lack of help that they may not see the problem either. More divisiveness can also happen between moms, based on the number of children they have. Regardless of whether a mother has one child or ten, postnatal care is important and impacts the health of the mother and the family.

A large part of acknowledgment of postnatal care is centered around the conversations about women's health and women's reproductive lives amongst women. These conversations can start at home between mothers, daughters, aunts, nieces, grandmothers, etc. Please be mindful that stories can offer practical and useful information. There's a lot we stumble upon as women, that if shared with each other could be tremendously helpful. I broach some of these topics in my blog, *Yoni Box*, which focuses on breaking past the taboos of women's reproductive health and perspectives and remedies to assist women naturally.

Check out a savvy blog by Dr. Danett on natural ways to enjoy good reproductive and overall health as for women.
http://yonibox.com

I knew some general principles of the importance of postnatal care from specializing in women's health for my doctorate in acupuncture and Asian medicine, and I understood a lot about women's health from specializing in it in my private practice for more than 12 years. But the truth is that I don't see many mothers in my practice, and those that I do see usually have older children. Still, there was so much that I didn't know about proper postnatal care, and my guess from informal research is that I am not alone. Many people do not know. But I think it starts with us, as women, acknowledging the importance of postnatal care and helping people who don't know.

What are the kinds of conversations that need to happen between women? I call these the 3 P's.

The 3 P's
1. Pleasant and Positive Experiences
2. Practical Things
3. Powerful Things

Pleasant and Positive Experiences
After just one person chose to delve into a horror birth story when I was pregnant, I started to wonder what was wrong with people. Of all the things you could share with an expecting mother, why that? This story haunted me for a while, but eventually I was able to delete the file from my brain (flooding my head with child birth stories from Ina May Gaskin also helped). The woman who shared her version of *Nightmare on Elm Street* (I guess that would be *Nightmare on Pregnancy Street*) was just looking for a way to heal her pain, because the story she told wasn't even about her own birth experience. The truth is, there are lots and lots of horror stories for each stage

of a woman's reproductive health. Why not "eliminate the negative and accentuate the positive?" If you hear a negative story about a woman's reproductive health, dump the negative aspects, extract only the useful parts, and pass that on. That brings us to the next P of practical things.

Practical Things

Many of us have very practical information that we just forget to share. For instance, a patient of mine happened to mention that she came across some information that many commercial sanitary pads have ingredients that can affect the body's chemistry, including hormones. I responded, "Oh you didn't know that?" And she exclaimed, "Dr. Bean! You've been holding out on me!" I said, "Sorry, I didn't realize you didn't know." In a similar way, I wish someone would've told me that when you potty train a boy, it's best if you start them sitting down so that urination and defecation can go into the potty, as opposed to having a proud-faced little one standing with poop on the floor behind him. Ah, it seemed to take forever to get him to sit down to poop. Practical information just makes things easier. So if you have practical information about any women's reproductive health topic, first be open to these conversations and then spread the wealth. The person who's listening will most likely be able to discern if it's for her, will do additional research, and will hopefully have more conversations about it. I think it is particularly important to share the information that you think everybody knows, because chances are there's someone who doesn't.

Powerful

I believe within each of us is our own unique connection to a higher power, source, or whatever you like to call it. So when you tell someone about a positive experience, it sends good energy. When you tell someone something practical, it's helpful. And when you tell someone something empowering, it resonates with an inherent strength that we are all waiting to act on. Too often between women, it can be all too easy to tear each other down—but we are the ones that get hurt. It's time to empower each other. The various stages of a woman's reproductive health can be times of being in tune with a greater power, which is extremely powerful. I've noted this to be particularly true during pregnancy. Remind women that they have a direct line to Source through their connection with, and as, the divine feminine. Every situation and woman is different, but generally a woman may not need a whole pep talk on what she's going through and her reproductive life. Rather, it seems to be extremely helpful to empower a woman by helping her remember what already exists within her. This will help her to remember her power. This is empowerment.

Positive, practical, and powerful conversations between women on women's healthcare set the stage to further educate each other about core issues, like postnatal care. Some suggestions come from my personal experience and will be scattered throughout the book, particularly in the chapters on support and practical steps to help a mother.

Sister circles and events like red tent circles are essential to restoring much-needed dialogue of the indigenous wisdoms of the feminine for all stages of womanhood, including post-natal care.

 Watch Video Interview with Mut Ra-t/Geralyn Heard-Harry on the importance of Red Tents in preventing postnatal depletion.
http://backtothemiddle.com/?p=1267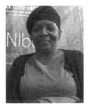

Mut Ra-t/Geralyn Heard-Harry is the founder of Red Tent Circle of Life!, a postpartum doula and has been working with mothers for over 40 years. She can be contacted at wombkeepers1@gmail.com.

General Public/ Good Ideas Travel Fast

From these conversations between women, information will hopefully naturally spread to the general public. Maybe not as fast as the latest celebrity gossip, but good ideas travel fast.

Education about the importance and details of postnatal care can be disseminated in conversations, some of which are not just between women. It's a great thing for boys and men to know how to help the women and future women that they love in their lives. If you are not a mother, when you come across one you can take a few minutes to genuinely ask her how she's doing? I think this is an important practice toward all human beings, but given the focus of this book on postnatal care, particularly toward mothers. You can ask her how her postnatal care is going. If she looks at you with a blank stare, you may need to teach her about postnatal care. Either way, be prepared to listen to her (acknowledgment), and as she has space this can help her to do the same with other mothers.

In general, the veil around women's reproductive health must be raised so that we can all see clearly and be able to help and strengthen all aspects of woman's reproductive health, including the postnatal care period. This time after giving birth is so important and so sacred that some are now terming it the fourth trimester. In her book, *Healing Your Body Naturally After Childbirth: The New Mom's Guide to Navigating the Fourth Trimester*, Dr. Jolene Brighten discusses the importance of this time, along with excellent remedies to assist new mothers. I very much wish it had been around when I was an expectant or new mom. Depending on the individual, a woman may need targeted health care for an even longer time, and assistance with her family on an ongoing basis.

Everyone needs to know about postnatal care, in hopes that it can be integrated or reintegrated into one's culture. Acknowledgement of postnatal care involves:

- Pregnant women
- Partners of pregnant women and those that hope to be a future partner of a pregnant woman
- Medical professionals that may interact with mothers and don't give full weight to the importance of postnatal care.

Each of the above members could be part of the postnatal community, which we will talk about next.

CHAPTER 4

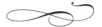

Community

Watch Video Message:
Danett C. Bean, DAAM Introduces Chapter 4
http://backtothemiddle.com/a-taste-of-our-own-medicine-book-chapter-4-introduction-video/

When I was pregnant and preparing for our new little one, I did everything I could think of to get ready for him. We got all of the sweet baby clothes, the perfect baby carrier, baby toys, and cloth diapers. We took a baby carrier class, a Bradley class, and learned how to use a cloth diaper. I also collected names of family and friends, along with times that they would be available, to try to have help around consistently and to spread the wealth, i.e., not having a bunch of people around one day and none the next. For the first month of my son's life in August, friends and family did visit, and boy did I look forward to those visits. I loved my time with my son, but I also loved the company and not being isolated. When September came, however, the majority of the visits stopped. Although this was clearly a bit construed, I had always thought that somehow once you had a baby, all of this help would magically show up and happily give you what was needed. But I soon learned that this was but a dream, that perhaps only existed in faraway places. In retrospect, I realize what I had hoped for was community.

What is community, and specifically the type that can help to strengthen postnatal care?

Community can be defined as "a group of people who live in the same area, or who have a common interest." We will focus on the latter definition. In the case of postnatal care, the common interest would be preserving and strengthening the mother so that she can be healthy as well as her child/children and family.

A postnatal community could be categorized as follows:

● The postnatal professional team
● "At-home" postnatal care assistance

The Postnatal Professional Community

Obstetricians/gynecologists and midwives are typically the best professionals to help facilitate the baby, secondary, of course, to the mother. These people have specific information about birth and practical things that need to happen for the mother, can check in with how things are going with the healing process, and can follow up on general wellness and postnatal symptoms, such as checking stitches after a cesarean or episiotomy. This group is typically extremely knowledgeable, but sometimes maintain very busy practices, and/or do not focus on the details that need to be in place to help strengthen postnatal care. Other obstetricians and midwives are on it, and provide a key part of the skeleton for the postnatal professional team.

Doulas

Doulas play such a key role. They can act as an intermediary between the medical practitioners and the family. Best of all, their full commitment is to the mother, her choices and comfort, the baby, and the family. Doulas can help in a variety of ways that may vary greatly before, during, and after birth. In my opinion, they are angels dressed as human beings, who can really be the hub of postnatal professional care. It is important to discuss the type of assistance that you'd like from your doula ahead of time. It is also important to be clear about the proximity of the doula to you, and the frequency of visits that they are able to provide. It can be hard to anticipate everything you may need in advance as a new mother, but do know that the details can make all of the difference. Doulas meet needs that ultimately strengthen postnatal care and make a good fit. Doulas of North America (DONA) is an excellent resource to find a doula in your area. Just go to https://www.dona.org/what-is-a-doula/find-a-doula/. Their vision statement is "A doula for every person who wants one."

I personally believe that having a doula can be essential in preventing postnatal depletion.

Watch video interview with
Chanel Porchia-Albert on the roles
that doulas can play as part of the
postnatal professional team
http://backtothemiddle.com/?p=1273

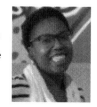

Chanel L. Porchia-Albert CD, CLC, CHHC is the Founding
Executive Director of Ancient Song Doula Services in Brooklyn,
New York and has received grants from Every Mother Counts
and the Foundation for the Advancement of Midwifery.
https://www.ancientsongdoulaservices.com

Additional Mother-Specific Therapists

Groups that offer specific therapies for mothers, like baby
and me yoga or lactation support groups, can be a very
important part of the postnatal care team, if the mother has
access to these resources. They have a specific and invaluable role, because these groups include other mothers. This
brings up another definition of community, which is "a feeling of fellowship with others." My favorite experience of this
was when I was pregnant and attended prenatal yoga class.
Honestly, other than the closeness I felt to my baby and how
I understand God, this was one of my favorite parts of being
pregnant. From my second trimester I attended weekly, often
two to three times a week until I was close to my due date.
Being around other mothers was priceless and helpful to my
labor. Many other organizations, like La Leche League and
The Mommies Network, offer support to mothers. Check our
directory of resources for more information. (See resource

section, Things That Personally Helped Me to Recover from Postnatal Depletion #12).

The "At-Home" Postnatal Care Team

If the mother has a partner, a good amount of the weight and responsibility will fall on them, particularly in many typical nuclear households in the United States. A partner may love the new mother intensely and just not have a clue of what to do. Hormonal changes, lack of sleep, the adjustment to a new life, the health of the family, finances, and more contribute to a complex situation which at best can put strain on a relationship. I can personally attest to this.

In certain ways, I believe my husband and I did well. For handling the basics with the baby, he would sweetly say that I handle the front (meaning nursing and pumping milk for the baby) and that he would handle the rear (meaning diaper changes and washing the cloth diapers). At bare bones, we worked together as a team to keep the basics going. Our focus and attention to the baby's needs was spot on, but our attention to each other's needs went out the window. I don't blame either one of us, as this was the result of many factors, but primarily I believe this was due to a lack of community and the resulting isolation. We were in survival mode, between the baby's needs, my sickness, keeping our businesses going, and paying the bills. It was like the weight of a huge bowling ball had come crashing down in the middle of a wooden table. It shook our foundation, rocked our core, and nearly broke the ties of a then almost decade-long relationship.

In the ideal setting we would have had more community, as would all parents. In addition to her partner, if the mother has one, she would also have other mothers around who are supported as well, and other welcomed people as part of the community. But while community is essential, the next topic is different than community, though they can sometimes be confused with one another. This is the crux of strengthening postnatal care: support.

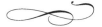

Support

Watch Video Message:

Danett C. Bean, DAAM Introduces Chapter 5

**http://backtothemiddle.com/a-taste-of-our-own-
medicine-book-chapter-5-video/**

Support can have many different definitions and associations, but the primary definition we will use is "to give assistance to." So we will be talking about support as an action, but also as a noun meaning "material assistance."

Acknowledgment that postnatal care exists is our first step in ending postnatal depletion/furthering postnatal care. This happens via conversations between women that contain the three P's: positive, practical, and powerful. This information would be disseminated through families and communities. People surrounding the mother would be aware of the importance of the postnatal time, with a conscious and clear common interest of preserving and strengthening the mother, so that the mother, the child/children, and the family would be nourished. Working together with a common interest would render them a community. The actions that the community would take is support.

I will make an important distinction here, which is that community doesn't necessarily equal support. You can have people gathered together, and as discussed in the last chapter generally have a common interest which makes them a community, but not necessarily know how to translate that common interest into support.

> "If the demand on a person grows, her resources should grow as well."
> **~Hanson, Hanson, & Pollycove, 2002**

It is important to note that we are talking about support as it could really be helpful to a mother, to help her to have more peace and a better physical and emotional state. With actual support, a mother could more easily pay attention to the things that help her to be sustained as she sustains the life/lives that are dependent on her. But please know, I have seen mothers with community but not support—meaning they had people with a common goal of helping, but without the action of helpfulness. In these cases, the "hypervigilance" that mothers can experience, which can lead to postnatal depletion, is not lessened (Serrallach, n.d .). Sometimes, community without support can contribute to postnatal depletion. For support to happen, it really comes back to "a taste of our own medicine." It is important to remember that essentially, mothers are the slabs of wood that form a foundation, and many times also fill the gaps. Support is anything that can help to fill the gaps, so that the mother doesn't have to spread herself thin.

How Do You Know What To Do?

You ask her. Many mothers are so accustomed to doing things themselves, they may not know how to answer, but give her a few minutes and she will probably come up with something. During my experience with postnatal depletion, the most accurate description of what life would be like postnatally, and was such a wonderful example of support, happened at my son's naming ceremony. One of my friends came late, which was perfect because I was able to dip with the baby without seeming rude, and enough people had left so that I didn't have to play host. She was a mother herself and said, "It's going to be hard and you're not going to get help, but while I'm here can I do something?" Before leaving she took out the garbage, just because she saw it needed to be done. It was such a dear, truthful, and helpful moment.

Support comes back to some of the examples of indigenous cultures that have a high quality of postnatal care. As mentioned, these models seem to mimic that which the mother is providing to the baby: sleep/rest, nutrition, and peace/solace. Let's explore further the importance of each of these, along with ways to help mothers get a taste of our own medicine.

Sleep/Rest

When my son was five months old, my midwife was worried that he wasn't gaining enough weight, so she referred me to a lactation consultant. The lactation consultant put us back on a newborn feeding schedule. While I was happy to help my son to get what I was told he needed, it was absolute hell, because we had just been getting into a rhythm of him sleeping through the night. Going back on the schedule helped him gain the weight that the consultant thought he needed, but it made me miserable. Sleep deprivation is a terrible thing. Nothing makes sense. Many mothers end up having to choose between eating or sleeping (occasionally a shower may be an option), but when you have to choose between two vital activities, you know you're in intense times. From my personal experience and research, going without sleep for long periods of time is the hardest thing about the postnatal period.

An excellent way to support a mom is to coordinate someone that the mom feels safe with to watch the baby, while she gets some rest. You can also offer to do some of the housework or errands that the partner would be doing, so that he is freed up to be with the baby or to do things that the mother may feel are too personal to ask. Restful sleep will always help the body to regenerate. From a traditional Asian medical standpoint, good quality sleep helps to improve the heart energy, which is closely connected with blood. In this system it is also believed that breast milk is a byproduct of blood, which is made during sleep. Sleep helps one to be in a better mood, and mood is such an important ingredient when caring for a new life.

Nutrition

"All mothers need to consciously replenish their lost nutritional and energetic reserves during the postpartum period. If this isn't done, they might end up spending the rest of their lives wondering why they 'just haven't felt the same since the baby was born.'"
~Dr. Dean Raffelock, 2008

After being sick for close to two years with varying illnesses postnatally, I prayed. I had so much pain and discomfort. I had seen some of the very best healthcare practitioners. Each was helpful in their own way, but I was still getting sick. For a while I was taking so many supplements that it was like my immune system existed in the bottles that I would pry open with tired, desperate hands.

Around my birthday I did something that I felt guilty about, but later came to realize was a great decision. I went for a short, under two-day stay to the Jersey shore. It was too cool for me to go into the water comfortably, but I knew that being by the ocean would help to restore me, as it always had. I made sure to have time where I did nothing on the trip, which wasn't easy because there were so many things I was behind on that I felt needed to be addressed. I also made certain to have time to go within.

I sat with myself, trying to figure out what I needed to get better. It took a while to sort out, and then finally it came to me: the soup! I had planned to make some special soup in my last trimester and freeze it, but, as I mentioned, we had to move unexpectedly. When we moved into the new place, I was in my last month of pregnancy. We moved in while the renovations were still being completed, and the kitchen was the last room to be renovated. There had been so much on my mind that I had forgotten the soup! I did recall there was a time since the labor that I had remembered it, but this memory was not totally clear, and it was muddled in my own longings for someone else to figure out. But they didn't figure it out, and it was up to me. I had some ideas from my Eastern nutrition background of what to put in the soup, but I did some more research. I knew it was going to help me. I made it weekly, took it consistently, and it played a major role in my healing. My son loved it and lapped it up too! (The recipe is included in the resources section). This magic soup included a whole chicken, bone broth (sorry to my vegan friends who didn't know I can sometimes be a closet carnivore, lol), and herbs. Bit by bit the soup regenerated my spirit and my blood, and brought me back to life.

My health issues weren't all solved, but I turned a big corner. While this recipe is not indigenous to my culture and may not be to yours, it was very, very helpful. Feel free to make this soup and/or share this recipe with any mother who is open to it. Trace your indigenous roots and see what foods were, and perhaps are still, used in your lineage to build back mothers, or ask others about their traditions, or do your own research.

One thing that is sometimes used by mothers or baby when ill is the placenta. It can be ground up and made into a tea or tincture. This is easy to get ahold of if you have a home birth. If you give birth in the hospital they may give you some trouble, but they have to give the placenta to you, as it is yours. In traditional Asian herbal medicine, we sometimes add placenta from an animal to an herbal formula, as it rebuilds *jing*, or essence, and strengthens *qi*, or energy, and blood. If you or someone you know is vegan and seeing an herbalist, another herb can be selected. Placenta, however, is a magic remedy that can help so many health issues, including postnatal depletion. Here are a few important things that I wish I would have known:

1. There are people that can encapsulate or make your placenta into a tincture, and most of us are better off having a professional do it. They will check to make sure that the placenta is viable. Some may even pick it up and drop it off to the mother.

2. If you think you may want to use your placenta, make sure you have room cleared out in your freezer. That's where you should store it until it's prepared.

3. And most importantly (which I wish someone would've told me), *the longer you wait to get the placenta prepared the more it loses its potency.* The people that I wanted to encapsulate my placenta informed me that six months is the maximum time that you can use a placenta from the time of the birth. After that you do have the option of using it for spiritual purposes and rituals, or doing something creative with it, like placenta art (Yup. Who knew?).

I knew in advance that I wanted to save and use my placenta, but I didn't know this other information, nor did I have a plan for how I would get it encapsulated. By the time that I had the mental clarity, the energy, and the ability to make it a priority, the placenta had expired past the point that it could've been used for internal medicinal purposes. Taking the placenta to get encapsulated could be the perfect job for someone who wants to help a mother but knows that they will be unable to be around a lot, or for the person who is like how I used to be—scared to hold a baby (my husband was like that too, although obviously we had to get over that, lol). This is something you may want to set up in advance and to include as part of your postnatal plan (See resource section, Postnatal Care Template Checklist).

Life happens and everything can't be planned, but having some ideas and help setting things up in advance can be invaluable. These plans can act like anchors on a boat that was once floating along unintentionally. The Postnatal Care Template Checklist is included to help serve as an anchor.

Whole foods are an essential ingredient in keeping the mother strong. Continuing postnatal vitamins at least through nursing, and/or as recommended by your health care professional, can also prove to be quite helpful. While I believe the most important place to get nutrition is through whole foods (assuming that the nutrients are being properly assimilated), two supplements that I personally found helpful were alfalfa tablets and Innate Response's Baby and Me Trimester III. Alfalfa, which is rich in minerals, can also help milk supply.

It's like nature's own multivitamin. I really liked using Innate Response's Baby and Me Trimester III because it is all whole foods-based, which means it's less foreign and easier for the body to digest. I have learned that the ingredients have been reformulated since I took it, so I can no longer vouch for the efficacy of this particular supplement. However, alfalfa tablets are still excellent. These supplements would be a great gift for a mom. There are companies that allow supplements to be shipped on a continuing monthly basis, such as Emerson Ecologics. You can cancel at any time.

Additional nutrients that some experts have cited as important postnatally are vitamins B (including B12), C, D, calcium, magnesium, alpha lipoic acid, coenzyme Q10, iron, zinc, and copper. Omega 3s have also been cited as important, and this nutrient personally made a huge difference in improving my health, including sharpening my cognition and making my skin healthier. It is best to seek a competent medical practitioner for appropriate guidance on this.

All of these things help the mother's body to stay at its healthiest and support the baby. Nutrition can be a very personal decision, particularly as it pertains to vegetarianism versus a diet that includes animals and animal byproducts. As someone who has utilized both diets, I believe that there are a multitude of factors that make a particular way of eating right for someone. From my personal and clinical research, I believe conscious eating is key, and that certain diets and foods are better depending on the life stage and resulting dietary needs of an individual.

Watch Video Interview with Nya Memaniye Cinque as she gives her perspective on nutritional advice for preventing and healing postnatal depletion.
http://backtothemiddle.com/?p=1271
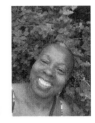

Nya Memaniye Cinque, CNM, NP is a certified nurse midwife of almost 20 years, nutritionist, and founder of Dyekora Sumda Midwifery in Brooklyn, New York.
http://www.dyekorasumda.com/.

Water

Now this one may sound just too simple, but before you chalk it up as a no-brainer consider these stories:

I was producing a pretty good milk quantity, but noticed sometimes during the day I'd feel more fatigued. A dear friend of mine and mother of four told me to always sit with a big cup of water and drink when I got ready to nurse. I tried it and noticed that not only did I not feel as tired after, I also produced more milk when I pumped.

Second story, years later I went to get some blood work done after I had just finished drinking a big cup of water. One nurse was like, "Wow, her blood is really flowing." The other nurse said, "That's because she just drank all that water." And there you have it, a perfect example of how water quickly and directly affects our body fluids.

Honestly, it can be all too easy to not drink enough water. Through surveying patients over the years, it seems that the majority of people do not drink enough water. Chronic dehydration is very, very common. This is important for all of us, but it is particularly important for a nursing mother. Water is vital to her well-being and can really support the mother in key ways if she is breast-feeding. Some tips that can help a nursing mother have a healthy water intake are:

1. Check in with the mother and ask about her water intake. Sometimes just asking someone about drinking water can help them to remember to do it. An additional benefit may be that you asking her will help you remember to drink more water, as well.

2. Bring the mother some water if you are with her when she is nursing or about to nurse.

3. Consider giving her a water-related gift. This can be interesting as there are all kinds of factors that can influence hydration habits. For example, some people may have a Brita, but may never remember to replace the filter. Or they may have misplaced their water bottle or live somewhere where it's hard to transport water up the stairs. Just asking about her water situation could be very helpful. You may decide to gift her with some method of water filtration, or a new water bottle, or have water delivered.

These are things that can seem simple, but can make a huge difference to the mother's physical health, overall mood, and milk supply for the baby. The next and last topic is just as vital but a bit more complicated: peace/solace.

Peace/Solace—The Antithesis of Stress

Peace/solace does wonders for health, but in this day and age it is all too easy to be stressed out. How many times has someone told you not to stress? It can be a nice gesture, but when stress is intertwined with basic needs, related to things that are on a deadline, or when things are challenging but must be done, peace/solace can be even more difficult to negotiate.

Not quite a month had passed since having my son when I got a letter that my health insurance was going to be cut. My son was good for a year, but I was not. As a friend of mine joked, "It's not like the baby needs someone to take care of him." I did my best to get in the necessary paperwork, but it ended up not being turned in by the deadline. Fortunately, a mother in the know told me about someone that could help me to reapply for insurance. I reapplied and was approved. That was practical help (one of the 3 p's) and almost instantly decreased my stress, leaving me feeling positive and powerful (the other 2 p's).

Stress can be such an interesting little (or enormous) bugger. From a traditional Asian medical standpoint, for good emotional and physical health, your *qi* (similar to energy) must be moving well through the body. Stress does the complete opposite, causing qi to stagnate. You may not always feel when your *qi* is stagnant, but some of the ways that this can manifest physically include headaches, bloating, irritability, and/or frustration. In traditional Asian medicine, the liver plays a key role in how stress is negotiated in the body. The liver channel passes through the breast, sometimes causing pain and masses to form. For nursing mothers, stress can totally affect milk production.

One mother I knew was producing milk just fine for her baby, until one of her parents—who should have been there to support her—kept telling the new mother that she was not capable of producing enough milk for the baby. Hearing this caused stress, and the mother's milk production actually lessened. How about that for irony? This brings us back to support. Support is essential in eliminating postnatal depletion, as it deepens the dimensions of postnatal care. It is important to remember that based on the relationship, it can be nice to have someone around, as company. But just because someone is around as community, this does not necessarily equal support. This story perfectly illustrates the need for support and community, the steps that can actually help to give a mother a taste of her own medicine. Having a community, along with the awareness to give mothers the support they need, can be a natural stress reliever.

Anyone and Everyone Can Make a Difference!

I'll say it again. Anyone and everyone can make a difference. That includes you. Yes you! You can make a difference here. From the person that has the time to be available to a mother for five minutes, an hour, a few hours, or a day, to the person who is unable to be around ever. It all comes down to four simple words that you can ask the mother in a variety of ways, "Do you need anything?", "How can I help? ", "Can I do something?" Sometimes people may feel afraid that they will be asked to contribute in a way that they can't or don't feel comfortable with. If you can't do what she's asked of you, just say you can't do it, but you'd still like to help. "What else can I do?" Okay that's five words, but you get my drift, lol. From my personal experience, it seems like sometimes people feel as though there are two extremes; that they can either give lots and lots, or nothing at all, but in reality that's not true. There is a huge spectrum in between. And honestly, the smallest gesture can make a mother's day, give her one less thing to worry about, and allow her a bit more room to share love, affection, and herself the way she'd really like to with her baby, child/children, and family. And after all, the baby feels everything the mother does, her joys and her stresses, without her saying a word.

Examples of ways to help if you are short on time:

1. Offering to pick up a few items from the grocery store.
2. Stopping by and putting out the garbage.
3. Mailing letters
4. Picking up some diapers or purchasing a diaper service
5. Helping with laundry

And the list goes on and on. I surveyed a group of mothers and came up with a list, "Specific Tips to Help Mothers", in the resource section. There are two things that I always do for mothers. First, whenever I see a mother nursing, whether I know her or not, I offer to bring her some water. At first, she'll resist, but eventually accepts and is always thankful that she did. She will often say that she hadn't been drinking enough water. The other thing I always do: if a mother hasn't eaten, I won't talk to her until she does. It's my modern day reverse Gandhi. For most mothers, they will never ignore the hunger of their child, but will so easily sacrifice their nutrients. There are places and situations where the mother may not have access to food, but in the situations I've experienced, many do have access. It seems to me that we've gotten so used to carrying on without, that we don't know when to stop and that it is not only important, but essential, that we get what we need.

If you have a close-enough relationship with a mother, and she feels comfortable, you could perhaps care for the baby for half an hour. This could do wonders. It's real in the mommy field. So chances are if you are available for 30 minutes (obviously you can offer more time if you have it), the mother will use that time extraordinarily well and be so appreciative. She may even choose to use it just to go outside and get some air. Which brings me to another precious tool that can bring peace/solace to the mother.

On my baby's first pediatric visit, the doctor said something very important. He said, "The most important thing you can do for the health of your baby", I remember feeling so excited, like he was about to impart some real jewel, which I was so desperate for, "is for you to get outside every day alone and take a walk by yourself." "What???", I thought to myself.

Honestly I wasn't thinking he'd say anything like that. The thought of it sounded so indulgent. I felt a little excited about getting some regular time to myself, and then a twinge of guilt passed through me. I did follow the doctor's orders and it was so helpful.

In the future, when postnatal care is more full and multidimensional, taking a regular walk alone as a mother might become standard, or maybe we'll figure out something totally different. In any event, we need additional proposals for the future, and that is just what the next chapter delves into.

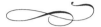

A Proposal for the Future

Watch Video Message:
Danett C. Bean, DAAM Introduces Chapter 6
http://backtothemiddle.com/a-taste-of-our-own-medicine-book-chapter-6-introduction-video/

Without question, furthering the depth of postnatal care is an essential element in eliminating postnatal depletion. While it has been estimated that the effects of postnatal depletion can last for up to 10 years, I suspect that the effects may extend beyond that (Serrallach, n.d.). Some women may develop various attitudes, emotions, and conditions during this time period that can affect the rest of their life. The work of a mother can be extremely physical. You are essentially the earth, house, supermarket, and security for a new life or lives. These responsibilities continue, and can take many forms as your children grow. As such, economic support, including paid leave and health insurance, is an essential starting point in developing a truly workable plan for postnatal care for mothers and families.

Paid Leave

Many places throughout the world provide parents with paid leave. I think this may be due to an understanding of the very important work that mothering is, and it is also simply human. Paid leave is vital for furthering postnatal care and the elimination of postnatal depletion. Here are some of the reasons why paid maternity and paternity leave should continue to be rallied for until it is a standard in the U.S.

1. It Lessens Stress

The number one stress for many of the families that I've spoken with is finances. It's interesting that the United States is currently one of the richest countries in the world, and still so many of us are stressed about money and so many are without. Lessening economic stress decreases stress on the mother, and that is obviously better for the baby. If you believe that the early experiences that a baby encounters affect their later life, then this is a very important reason.

2. It's Just Human

To make a mother and family have to choose between providing the vital things that only she can provide (familiarity, scent, breast milk, etc.) and returning to work prematurely to keep food on the table and provide a roof over their heads is ridiculous.

3. Returning to Work Prematurely Should Be Contraindicated for Anyone Who Is Still Ill

Preventing postnatal depletion is no different. Without adequate rest and nourishment, the likelihood of postnatal depletion occurring most likely increases. This can lead to additional health complications and consequently increase health costs in the long run.

4. It's Just Good

It's good for the child to have a relaxed parent. When basic resources are covered, stress goes down and health is better. Having paid leave would help to make sure the basics are covered.

Insurance

1. Insurance that extends through the first year after giving birth, without requiring renewal, would be very helpful for new mothers. It can be challenging enough adjusting to a new life as a mom, coupled with health visits for the child and the mother. Let's not give the mother one more thing to do.

2. Given that postnatal depletion affects an estimated 50% of mothers and can have long- lasting effects, making sure that mothers are insured is key.

3. After giving birth, mothers are typically focusing on and adjusting to life as a mother. The expectation to get paperwork in so soon is an unnecessary burden.

4. It is extremely important that babies and children have someone who is healthy to take care of them. It makes sense that mothers maintain the basics that they need to help them to be able to function for this very important job. Keeping mothers insured just makes sense.

The night that I discussed at the beginning of the book, which was one of many in which I didn't know where I was, happened after work. I had been with my baby during the day, taught a class that evening, and then pumped. Because I was already very blood-deficient, primarily from the significant amount of blood loss I'd had during labor, and because I hadn't built myself back up, I literally had nothing else to give by the end of the night. Under a different economic system, one that recognizes the value and work of mothers and parents, I, like many other women, would not have had the need to return to work so quickly and unintentionally risked my life. Incidentally, the Family and Medical Leave Act (FMLA) allows twelve work weeks of leave in a 12-month period for eligible employees, which is a luxury for those who don't have this option. However, a 2011 study by Dr. Julie Wray, in which she interviewed mothers in the first year of postnatal life, revealed that they needed one year off to recuperate physically and emotionally.

Models from Around the World

Many cultures around the world have historically understood, and continue to understand, the importance of the postnatal care time. It is interwoven within the fabric of the society, as the intrinsic value of producing another human being and the respect and care that is required is understood. In the interim, as the awareness of postnatal care hopefully spreads, postpartum recovery centers are needed. The first of these centers is said to have started in Beijing, China. Here in New York, there are ten professional postpartum centers that I've learned of (there may be more that have not been documented). These centers are mainly run out of apartments in Flushing and Bayside, Queens, with the monthly cost of a program ranging anywhere from $3,000-$5,000. Perhaps someday soon, such programs will be seen as a necessary component of care, and the entire cost will not have to come out of the pocket of the family. Though to some this may sound costly, I don't believe it to be more costly than the cost of health care for the effects of untreated postnatal depletion. This is key, particularly to families who are without support. I believe that true preventive care is always less costly in the long run, not only financially, but for the body, mind, and spirit.

The Truth

The truth is that in the 21st century, in the United States, capitalism is our current economic structure. While it provides lots and lots of benefits and has improved quality of life for many, there are ways that it hasn't benefited us. The average number of work hours for people ages 25–54 holding full-time jobs is 42.8 weekly. In addition to hours worked at the job, many people bring home work, and then there are the requirements just to stay on top of the many emails, and other responsibilities for those with and without families. This can make the natural activity of communities spending time together even more challenging. For many of us, work and personal obligations interfere with leisure time, time to take care of one's self, and time to express one's talents, let alone finding the time to play more of a role within family life or community.

Final Thoughts

With an estimated one out of two women dealing with postnatal depletion, something needs to shift to end this. First, we must have awareness that such a thing exists, along with community and real support for mothers. Since going through my own experience and writing this book, I've encountered numerous mothers who, through dialogue, realize that they may have, or have had, postnatal depletion. That it may not have been depression, or that what was going on was not just in their head, but that they may have had or currently have an actual physical health condition. For many, it was a relief to realize that it wasn't just them individually having a hard time, but a syndrome that affects a number of women.

Without question, I believe that there is strength in education and action, especially when we take it upon ourselves to be the ones to make a difference. I hope that this writing serves some role in furthering awareness and education of postnatal depletion, so that it can end. As best I see, gently and without blame, keeping our bodies healthy prior to and regardless of conception is important. Having community and support systems in place is important for all of us, but in particular these are essential ingredients for the care of a mother after giving birth, and throughout the experience of motherhood. Many of us have struggled and "made it", without it, but the question is: should we?

The role that mothers play is often the foundation of the household, but it also extends far beyond that to each and every crevice of the world. Do we want anyone not in good health, giving more than they have to, to keep things afloat? Sadly, I reflect on the mothers I know that have passed before even the age of 60. And after going through my own experience and talking with other mothers, I wonder if postnatal depletion, it's effects, and perhaps the mechanisms that were learned to struggle on, contributed to what I believe was premature passing. The work of making another human being can seem to happen easily and effortlessly in the body, but still requires support. Let us have dialogues on these topics, and learn what we can from the indigenous cultures who have maintained their reverence for the divine work of motherhood and the respect and care that it deserves with emphasis on the mother, not just during the prenatal period but afterwards as well.

With love and light,
Dr. Danett

Resources
Section

For the Mother Who Thinks She May Have Postnatal Depletion

Dear Mother,

How are you? I mean, how are you really doing? Though we most likely do not know each other, I hope that you are well and getting the support that you need to make your life really work. If you are feeling well, that is great, carry on with what you are doing and share what has helped you with other mothers and those that may become mothers. The things that you and mothers like you have figured out are invaluable to all our well-being. If, however, you are not feeling well, or have felt like something isn't quite right, you are not alone.

While the main postpartum condition that many of us in the United States hear about is depression, postnatal depletion is also a common condition, though from my research, it often goes undiagnosed. Postnatal depletion can contribute to postpartum depression and vice versa. Symptoms can include, but are not limited to, low energy, poor memory, and forgetfulness. I myself experienced a weakening of my joints and intense changes in my immune system. If you have experienced any of these signs, or have had health conditions that have surfaced and become chronic since giving birth, you may have postnatal depletion.

Please know that you are not alone. Many of us have felt the pressure that something is wrong with us if we don't just snap back into shape and get back to business as usual. If you have felt like you are crazy, most likely you are not, you may just be depleted. The great thing is that help and resources are available. Your next step is to seek the necessary assistance so that you can be replenished and feel better again. I went through a huge bout of postnatal depletion for years, and while I am still on the road to maintaining my health, I can say it is possible to get better. Please check our directory for potential practitioners and resources in your area. If you do not find any, I work with mothers virtually. You can find my contact information in the directory.

If you can decide to make and keep your health a priority (regardless of the guilt or other feelings that you may experience) and take consistent actions regarding your health, the way you would if it was your child, you are on your way to better health. For me, the only joy that I've experienced that is better than being a mother is being able to do so with better health and from a genuinely full cup. Take a deep breath, a better life may be closer than you think.

With love and light,
Dr. Danett

Specific Tips to Help Mothers

1. If you are a mother, share practical wisdom with other mothers and future mothers.

2. Tell only pleasant stories and say positive things about birth to a pregnant woman. Kindly remind her of the powerful state that she is in.

3. When you're going to the grocery store, ask if she needs anything and offer to drop it by her.

4. Offer gifts that are for the mother, not just for the baby or child. These can include a supply of the postnatal vitamins of her choice, drinking water related items (such as a bottle or filtration system), and gift cards so that she can pamper herself. A diaper service can also be really helpful to the mother and whole family.

5. Drop off food, including healthy prepared meals.

6. Arrange a time that works for you both when you can stop by and see if she needs anything. It could be for a few

minutes, hours, or a day. If both of you are comfortable, offer to be with the baby while she rests, showers, eats, or does whatever she needs. You can also offer to help do something that the partner is doing, or would do, so that they can be with the baby and the mother gets to do what she needs to.

7. See if there are errands that she needs assistance with. There may things you can do to help her without even coming to her house, especially if you are limited on time or she does not live close by.

8. If this is not the mother's first child, offer to watch the older sibling, or offer to spend time with the baby so she can spend one-on-one time with the older sibling(s).

9. If the mother has a partner, communicate to them how helpful the alone time is for the mother.

10. Offer to take a picture of the mother and her family. She may not be thinking of it now, but it's very likely that she will later realize she wished to have those moments captured.

11. Offer to do her laundry.

12. Compliment the mother by telling her what a great job she is doing.

13. When you visit her home, visit with the presence of peace.

Postnatal Care
Template Checklist

	Task	Notes
☐	**1. Diapers**	
☐	• Service will be provided by	
☐	• Purchased cloth diapers	
☐	• Will use disposable diapers	
☐	**2. Placenta Preparation**	
☐	• Will be provided by	
☐	• Placenta will be dropped off by	
☐	• Placenta will be picked up by	
☐	**3. Postnatal Professional team**	
☐	Midwife	
☐	Lactation Consultant	
☐	Other Therapist on hand (Acupuncturist, Massage Therapist)	
☐	**4. Core at Home Team**	
☐	• Doula (hours of availability, how long she will be available for)	
☐	• Back up doula	

	Task	Notes
☐	**5. Family and/or Friends that can come by to help**	
☐	Names and telephone numbers	
☐	*Doodle will be created by	
☐	**6. Mothers I can Call**	
☐	**7. Social Groups With Other Mothers**	
☐	Mommy friends to do play dates with	
☐	Mommy & Me Classes	
☐	Local Groups	
☐	Online Groups	
☐	**8. Social (Core Team Time)**	
☐	Regular time slots, even if brief	
☐	By Myself	
☐	With Partner	
☐	**9. Personal Care Items I need for myself**	
☐	**10. Online Grocery List and Passwords, Person who can do shopping**	
☐	**Anything I'd like to remember in case I forget**	

You can also access the Postnatal Care Template here

http://backtothemiddle.com/ postnatal-care-checklist-freebie/

List of Key Things That Personally Helped Me to Recover from Postnatal Depletion

1. Chicken Herb Soup
Nourish Blood and Essence Soup

1 ounce Dioscorea root (*Shan Yao*)
2 ounces Lycii berries (*Gou Qi Zi*)
1 ounce Lotus seeds (*Lian Zi*)
12 Red Dates (*Dao Zao*)—soaked and pitted
2 cups chopped greens (kale, chard, spinach, etc.)
7 cups chicken or bone soup stock
1 yam, diced
5 black or shitake mushrooms, slivered (if dry, soak first)
1/4 cup rice wine or rice vinegar

Break dioscorea into small pieces and simmer in soup stock along with the lycii berries and lotus seeds for 1 hour.
Add *dao zao*, yam, and mushrooms and simmer for another 20 minutes.

Add rice wine and greens and cook for 5 more minutes. Serve hot.

Courtesy of the Jade Institute, compilation by Cindy Micleu available online at: https://www.jadeinstitute.com/jade/post-partum-care-optimal-health.php

To order herbs for this soup, please email info@backtothemiddle.com

2. Moxibustion

Moxibustion is a part of traditional Asian medicine and a technique often used by acupuncturists. It is the process by which an herb is heated and placed over specific areas of the body. An acupuncturist can best show you how to do this, as well as which placement is best for you given your health issues.

3. Flents Quiet Please Ear Plugs

I have been able to experience a deeper sleep with ear plugs. I can still hear my child; it just helps to block out less significant noises that would wake me since I became such a light sleeper after becoming a mom.

*Please make sure to keep them out of reach of little ones.

4. *Flavored Water*

I lost a lot of blood in labor, and building back my blood and body fluids was a very important part of my recovery. Drinking water is so important, but sometimes the plain taste is not appealing. Naturally flavoring my water with slices of orange, lemon, goji berries, and apple helped me to fall back in love with water again and rehydrate. Goji berries are a favorite herb of mine.

Watch video with Dr. Danett on why Goji
berries are a girls best friend!
**http://backtothemiddle.com/
gojis-are-a-girls-best-friend/**

5. *Taking It Slow*

This is easier said than done, but was very helpful during my recovery.

6. *Louise Hay's* Self Healing, *listened to during naps.*

7. *Acupuncture*

Both my husband and I are licensed acupuncturists, so as long as neither of us were too tired (which was a lot of the time), I was able to get treatments. If you live in the New York area, my practice is currently in Brooklyn, NY, and at the time of this writing I'm still taking patients. You can find my contact information in the resources directory as well as other practitioners.

8. Yoga

Yoga is/was a lifesaver for me. I am a big fan of any of the healing disciplines that help one to slow down and unite breath, intention, and action. This includes Qi Gong and Tai Chi.

Access *5 Minutes of Energetic Recharge For Total Women's Health* here
http://backtothemiddle.com/5-minutes-of-energetic-recharge-for-total-womens-health-video/

9. Walks in the Park and Earthing

Earthing is connecting to the Earth's energy through skin contact.

10. Help from My Husband and Doula

Having a good close squad who can help you carry out your mission is priceless. Once we got a doula, it was immediately and deeply helpful for my family. It took some pressure off my husband and I, and allowed us to start to really see each other again.

11. Nordic Naturals Pro EFA

I like this company because they have good quality products and excellent testing standards to make sure there are no heavy metals in their products. They also have a supplement specifically designed for the postnatal period called Postnatal Omega 3.

12. A Host of Amazing Health Practitioners
(See Resources Directory).

Access the Resources Directory here:
http://backtothemiddle.com/?p=1326

About the Author

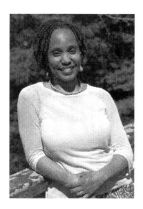

Dr. Danett C. Bean (Doctor of Acupuncture and Asian Medicine), affectionately called Dr. Danett, is a caring and compassionate healer who began studying health in the early nineties. Since then, she has become certified, licensed, and skilled in a variety of health disciplines and has administered thousands of treatments to assist people toward achieving better health. Though Dr. Danett's clinical experience is vast, her biggest health lesson came after having her son. Dr. Danett battled health conditions for years that almost took her life, but she survived victoriously and became passionate about spreading awareness on postnatal depletion. This resulted in the authoring of her book, *A Taste of Our Own Medicine: 3 Vital Keys to Ending Postnatal Depletion, Nurturing Mothers and Improving Our Communities.*

Dr. Danett identifies how postnatal depletion and other conditions can adversely affect women's health, both short-term and long-term. As such, she is dedicated to the essential practice of proper preventive care for women. This intersection of preventive care and women's health is where Dr. Danett feels most passionate, and is why she continues to be a fierce advocate for ending postnatal depletion and other conditions that can potentially be avoided. This passion fueled the creation of *Yoni Box*, a health-savvy blog that serves to break the taboos related to women's reproductive health and provide nature-based perspectives and solutions. Dr. Danett has also authored *Fibroid Prevention Guide*. In addition, she offers natural remedies that can support women, young and old, through key transitions in life. Dr. Danett lectures on this intersection of preventive care and women's health at various events. Additionally, Dr. Danett has created initiatives to support mothers, including a weekly support group for mothers and wives (currently closed) and the Yoni Box Annual 21 Day Mother's Day Challenge.

In her private practice, Dr. Danett assists women with the full spectrum of reproductive health concerns, including menstrual cycle issues for teenagers and adults, fertility readiness, labor preparation, postnatal care, hormonal imbalances, and menopausal symptoms. Dr. Danett uses herbal medicine, lifestyle recommendations, acupuncture, and other healing modalities via her signature Back To The Middle Method. This method addresses healing on a root level that aligns the body, mind, and spirit for optimal health. As an integrative medicine practitioner, who strongly believes in patient-centered medicine, Dr. Danett works with Western medical doctors and practitioners of various disciplines to best assist patients. Currently, Dr. Danett sees patients by appointment in her Crown Heights, Brooklyn office and offers virtual consultations to patients across the United States and all over the world.

Dr. Danett has a doctoral Asian medicine specialization in women's health and geriatrics, with a Diplomate of Asian Medicine. A New York state licensed acupuncturist, Dr. Danett is certified in Chinese herbology, eastern nutrition, and Earth Qi Gong for women. She is also a Clinical Instructor in the Department of Medicine at SUNY Downstate Medical Center and is appointed to the medical staff of the University Hospital of Brooklyn. Dr. Danett is also an adjunct professor in obstetrics and gynecology at Pacific College of Oriental Medicine, New York City. A former member of the medical staff of the Women's Health Center Empowerment Division at Housing Works and assistant producer of *Global Medicine Review*, Dr. Danett has helped organize community health expos including collaborations with the Caribbean Cultural Center African Diaspora Institute (CCCADI), WBAI, and Baruch College. She also has been a featured guest on radio and television media. Currently residing in Brooklyn, New York, Dr. Danett is a mother and wife.

References

Brighten, J. (2015). Healing your body naturally after childbirth: The new mom's guide to navigating the fourth trimester. Portland, Oregon: Brighten Wellness.

Childbirth Connection: A Program of the National Partnership for Women & Families (2017). What health concerns do U.S. women have after giving birth? A listening to mothers III data brief. Retrieved March 3, 2017 from http://transform.childbirthconnection.org/reports/listeningtomothers/healthconcerns/

Darwish, D.D. (2013, June 22). The working mothers' syndrome. *Strides.* Retrieved September 22, 2016 from https://coachingur3ps.wordpress.com/2013/06/22/the-working-mothers-syndrome/

DeCherney, A., Nathan, L., Goodwin, T.M., Laufer, N., & DeCherney, A.H. (2006). Current diagnosis & treatment obstetrics & gynecology (10th edition). New York, NY: McGraw Hill.

Doyle, A. (2016, November 14). What is the average hours per week worked in the US? *The Balance.* Retrieved April 3, 2017 from https://www.thebalance.com/what-is-the-average-hours-per-week-worked-in-the-us-2060631

Einhorn, A. (2001). The fourth trimester and you thought labor was hard: Advice, humor, and inspiration for new moms. New York, NY: Crown Publishers.

Hanson, R., & Hanson, J. (2007). Taking good care of moms. *New Beginnings*, 24(6), 274-275. Retrieved March 30, 2017 from http://www.lalecheleague.org/nb/nbnovdec07p274.html 3/30/17

Hanson, R., Hanson, J., & Pollycove, R. (2002). Mother nurture: A mother's guide to health in body mind and intimate relationships. London, UK: Penguin Books.

Hodnett, E.D., Gates, S., Hofmeyr, G.J., & Sakala, C. (2012, October 17). Continuous support for women during childbirth. *Cochrane Database of Systematic Reviews*. doi: 10.1002/14651858.CD003766.pub4

Hou, A.D. (2014, March 18). Sitting the month in Queens. *Open City*. Retrieved September 29, 2016 from http://opencitymag.com/sitting-the-month-a-new-take-on-a-chinese-tradition/

Housos, D. (2014, June 22). Pregnancy, birth, postpartum in different cultures—student article. *Birth Arts International*. Retrieved April 3, 2017 from http://www.birtharts.com/pregnancy-birth-post-partum-in-different-cultures-student-article/

Klewja, N. (n.d.). Postpartum rest and recovery tips (from a mama who learned the hard way). *Keeper of the Home*. Retrieved March 21, 2017 from http://www.keeperofthehome.org/postpartum-rest-and-recovery-tips-from-a-mama-who-learned-the-hard-way

Laing, K. (2015, August 21). How long does it really take to recover from pregnancy and birth? *Huffington Post*. Retrieved March 21,

2017 from http://www.huffingtonpost.co.uk/karen-laing/post-baby-body_b_8739254.html

Lee, H.J. (2013, January 25). Korean postpartum care is special. *Korea Times*. Retrieved September 15, 2016 from http://m.koreatimes.co.kr/phone/news/view.jsp?req_newsidx=129458

Maciocia, G. (1998). Obstetrics and gynecology in chinese medicine. London, UK: Churchill Livingstone.

Postpartum exhaustion (n.d.). *Berkeley Parent's Network*. Retrieved September 15, 2016 from https://www.berkeleyparentsnetwork.org/advice/pregnancy/exhaustion

Pregnancy and birth: Depression after childbirth – what can help? (2016, September 21). *PubMed Health/Informed Health Online*. Retrieved April 3, 2017 from https://www.ncbi.nlm.nih.gov/pubmedhealth/PMH0072762/

Raffelock, D. (2008). How pregnancy depletes nutrients. *Well Postpartum*. Retrieved March 21, 2017 from https://momswellness.wordpress.com/2008/12/30/how-pregnancy-depletes-nutrients/

Raffelock, D., Rountree, R., Hopkins, V., & Block, M. (2002). A natural guide to pregnancy and postpartum health: The first book by doctors that really addresses pregnancy recovery. New York, NY: Penguin Putnam.

Romm, A.J. (2002). Natural health after birth: The complete guide to postpartum wellness. Rochester, Vermont: Healing Arts Press, Inner Traditions International.

Ruiz, R. (n.d.). No family left behind. *Mashable*. Retrieved
    April 12, 2017 from http://mashable.com/2015/01/25/
    maternity-leave-policy-united-states/#FAnXVfRxhkq1

Serrallach, O. (n.d.). Postnatal depletion. Retrieved April 3, 2017
    from http://goop.com/postnatal-depletion-even-10-years-later/

The best thing about postpartum care in Germany (2016, July 26).
    Let the Journey Begin: Diary of a Trilingual Family. Retrieved
    September 15, 2016 from https://www.letthejourneybegin.eu/
    postpartum-care-germany/

U.S. Department of Health and Human Services' Office on Women's
    Health (2008). The healthy woman: A complete guide for all ages.
    Retrieved April 3, 2017 from https://www.womenshealth.gov/
    publications/our-publications/the-healthy-woman/

U.S. Department of Labor (2012). Fact sheet #28: The Family and
    Medical Leave Act. Retrieved April 12, 2017 from
    https://www.dol.gov/whd/regs/compliance/whdfs28.pdf

Wiseman, N., & Ellis, A. (1996). Fundamentals of Chinese medicine.
    Brookline, MA: Paradigm Publications.

Wray, J. (2011). *Bouncing back? An ethnographic study exploring the
    content of care and recovery after birth through the experiences and
    voices of mothers* (Doctoral thesis). Retrieved April 3, 2017 from
    https://www2.rcn.org.uk/_data/assets/pdf_file/0008/459035/
    Wray_Julie_complete_thesis_2011.pdf

Made in the USA
Columbia, SC
05 January 2020

86328927R00048